Revolutionizing Fitness

Women Influencers Transforming the Industry

Kate Virginia Todd

Table of Contents

I always did something I was a little not ready to do. I think that's how you grow. When there's that moment of 'Wow, I'm not really sure I can do this,' and you push through those moments, that's when you have a breakthrough.

— Marissa Mayer

Chapter 1. Introduction

Welcome to our Special Report: "Revolutionizing Fitness: Women Influencers Transforming the Industry". Immerse yourself in an inspiring, energizing journey of change led by women who are reshaping the fitness industry. Braced with determination, positivity, and raw grit, these ladies are proving that fitness is a realm open for all, where diversity thrives, and strength is the new definition of beauty. Encompassing powerful narratives, groundbreaking business endeavors, and entrepreneurial brilliance, this report promises an eye-opening deep dive into the fitness revolution that's shaking our world. Prepare to be captivated - this report is not just a read, but an experience that may make a profound impact on how you perceive fitness, strength, and the incredible power of women who dare to shake things up!

Chapter 2. The Pioneers: Women Who Broke Fitness Barriers

This segment of our Special Report delves into the rich histories and inspiring journeys of pioneering women who radically challenged, and subsequently revolutionized, the fitness industry. Embarking on daunting voyages of self-discovery and remaining resolute through adversity, these extraordinary women have shattered fitness stereotypes, emerging as genuine innovators in their sphere. They envisioned a world where fitness was not just for the elite or confined by gender, but rather, an inclusive realm that welcomed diversity, celebrated strength, and championed overall well-being.

2.1. The Birth of Women's Fitness: Early Trailblazers

To begin our exploration into the world of fitness pioneers, one must turn the pages of history. This brings us to Pudgy Stockton, dubbed the "First Lady of Iron," and Bonnie Prudden, a forward-thinking fitness guru. Both women made significant strides in an era that to some extent, resisted the idea of women engaging in intense physical fitness.

Stockton, in the 1940s, led the charge in getting women to train with weights. A witness to the transformative power of strength training, she defied societal barriers and established the Miss Physical Culture Venus pageant, a platform that celebrated women's musculature rather than typically idolized frailty. Stockton's Santa Monica Muscle Beach parties were further instrumental in carving a space for women in weightlifting and bodybuilding culture - a feat truly ahead of its time.

On the other hand, Bonnie Prudden, during the 1950s, highlighted the significance of physical fitness to overall health and well-being. Troubled by the low national fitness standards, especially among women and school children, Prudden developed a diagnostic system known as the 'Prudden Myotherapy'. This holistic fitness program promised to enhance muscle strength and flexibility as well as relieve pain through exercise.

2.2. Leap into the Twentieth Century: Diversification and Democratization

Advancing into the late twentieth century, the fitness industry saw a surge of women who changed the landscape even further. Jane Fonda, nicknamed "Queen of the Workout," heavily influenced the industry by launching an exercise video empire. Shaping the fitness fashion trends and introducing a whole new era of home workouts, Fonda brought fitness right into our living rooms.

Parallelly, Kathrine Switzer courageously broke barriers in the world of endurance sports. In 1967, she defied unspoken rules by registering and completing the Boston Marathon, an event hitherto open only to men. Her achievement was instrumental in prompting the inclusion of a women's marathon in the Olympics, forever changing endurance sports dynamics.

Around the same time, entrepreneur and weightlifter Betty Weider played an instrumental role in veering women's fitness away from just weight loss towards a robust focus on strength training. Through her magazine, 'Shape,' she confronted and changed the perception of women in fitness, emphasizing that health, strength, and shape – not just slimness - should be a woman's fitness destination.

2.3. Heralding the New Millennium: The Rise of the Fitness Rockstars

The new millennium saw the evolution of fitness mavens into celebrities in their own right. For instance, Jillian Michaels, of 'The Biggest Loser' fame, leveraged media to promote an empowering message. Michaels's idea of fitness was not about attaining a certain dress size; instead, she championed the idea that healthy living was a combination of physical wellness and mental strength.

Simultaneously, Michelle Bridges transformed the Australian fitness industry with her 12WBT (12 Week Body Transformation) programme. Bridges brought practicality and affordability center stage in fitness, showing that it was not the privilege of a few but achievable by all.

Through this chapter, we hope readers gain a profound respect for the pioneers who blazed trails in the fitness industry, paving the way for an inclusive present where opportunities abound. Their stories continue to inspire countless women worldwide, embodying the spirit of perseverance, innovation, and above all, the power of being pioneers in a conventionally male-dominated field. Truly, the fitness world of today owes a debt to the indomitable women who dared to challenge norms and revolutionize the fitness landscape.

Chapter 3. Evolving Fitness Ideals: The Shift Toward Strength and Well-being

In the vast tapestry of human history, the concept of beauty and its exemplifications have experienced vast transformations, transmuting as human society itself evolved. Paralleling these shifts, the realm of fitness has also witnessed significant metamorphoses in its ideals. Nowadays, there is a palpable sea change, where antiquated body image expectations targeted at women have been challenged and refuted, giving way to a buoyant wave of body positivity and a redefined focus on strength and well-being.

3.1. From Objectification to Empowerment

The earlier definitions of fitness were tightly interwoven with the very aesthetic image of the female body—a repository for societal objectification—serving no gratifying purpose to the women themselves. Squirming under the weight of these distorted expectations, women were coerced to strive for fitness goals that were more often than not, unattainable and perilous to their overall health.

However, as the winds of change began to blow, women stood against these constraints, choosing to transform the narrative. They recognized the urge to overthrow the existing standards of beauty and fitness, fighting against the regimented perceptions of physical attractiveness. Encapsulating the idea of empowerment, the new fitness aspiration for women became a holistic balance of toned and healthy bodies, robust mental health, and a strong spirit.

3.2. Strength: The New Beauty

In the heart of this evolution, strength assumed the mantle of the new aesthetic goal. The lopsided obsession with thinness made way for the broader concept of strength—embracing both physical power, as well as mental resilience. More important than the number on the scale, strength weaved itself into women's definition of fitness, emphasizing proper form, technique, endurance, and progressive growth.

This reimagining of the fitness landscape was no ordinary transformation; it became a passage for women toward self-affirmation, body acceptance, and liberation from societal impositions. Fitness was no longer an end, but a means— a journey to explore their potential, a narrative of personal victories, and quiet defiance.

3.3. The Rise of Well-being

On the other side of the fitness equation, an amplified focus on overall well-being has started to shape the industry. As awareness about mental health, nutritional balance, and the advantages of a positive lifestyle seeped into societal consciousness, fitness evolved to encompass these facets.

Fitness enthusiasts now strive to create a harmonious blend of physical fitness, mental health, and nutrition. They understand the importance of rest, stress management, and a balanced diet in addition to their exercise regimen. Fitness professionals worldwide are integrating mindful practices such as yoga, meditation, and breathwork into their fitness programs, acknowledging the critical interplay between the body and the mind.

3.4. Breakthroughs in Fitness Approaches

Complementing these paradigm shifts are innovations in training methodologies. Long gone are the days of tedious, monotonous workout routines. Today's fitness landscape brims with a plethora of training styles and programs, inspired by different sports and traditions, offering accessibility and options for women of all fitness levels.

These modern practices range from high-intensity interval training (HIIT) to functional training, flexibility-focused pilates to calm yoga sessions, hardcore crossfit to dance-based aerobic workouts. This diversity encourages women to choose what aligns with their fitness objectives, promoting adherence and love for the process, rather than just the results.

3.5. The Enthralling Potential of This Evolution

The reframing of fitness ideals has unleashed the unbounded potential within women. It has nurtured a new generation of trainees and influencers who are eager to shatter prevalent stereotypes and defy convention. This evolution points to a promising future where fitness is no longer a cage of societal expectations but a mode for women to express their strength, their resilience, their power, and ultimately, their invincible spirit.

The empowering narrative of strength and well-being inspires women worldwide to navigate their unique fitness journey, skillfully bypassing societal pressures and expressing their agency and autonomy. This thoughtful reconfiguration of fitness ideals is a compelling testament to the ever-evolving dynamism of the fitness industry and its powerful potential to transform lives, one workout at a time.

Chapter 4. Profiles of Power: In-depth Interviews with Leading Fitness Influencers

Let's begin our exploration into the lives and achievements of some truly inspiring women who have taken the fitness world by storm. We will take a deep dive into their backgrounds, their motivations, their training regimens, their philosophies, and, most notably, how they inspire and influence countless followers across the globe to pursue fitness as a lifestyle.

4.1. The Mettle Behind the Mascara: Alexandra Williams

An undisputed queen of fitness, Alexandra Williams fashionably jogs through the converging paths of fitness and modern femininity. With a sparkling career in elite-level fitness training, Williams has consistently broken stereotypes while promoting an inclusive understanding of fitness. Born and raised in Sydney, Australia, she developed an early love for sports but noticed a lack of representation for women. Her desire to change this narrative cultivated into a lifelong commitment to fitness. Today, her unique workout methodologies, seamless transitions between intense calorie burners to mindful yoga sessions, have gained worldwide recognition, motivating thousands around the world to start and continue their fitness journeys.

4.2. The Iron Rose: Jessica Ennis-Hill

Jessica Ennis-Hill, renowned Olympic gold medalist, is an epitome of power, demonstrating a unique blend of athletic prowess and tenacity. A native of Sheffield, England, Ennis-Hill's journey is one of enduring commitment and overcoming personal adversity. Despite facing various injuries throughout her career, this iron-willed woman has sculpted her mind and body into a formidable vessel of athletic performance. Her ethos of resilience in the face of adversity inspires millions globally, instilling the positivity needed to continue the quest for personal fitness goals.

4.3. Paving the Way for Progress: Mariana Pajón

Colombia's Mariana Pajón, a two-time Olympic gold medalist BMX racer, is an enduring beacon of inspiration for young women. Pajón's powerful strides on the BMX track are indicative of a bigger leap - towards equality in a typically male-dominated sport. With engaging narratives around her training sessions, diets, and tournament preparations, Pajón has amassed a dedicated following, significantly inspiring increased participation of women in extreme sports and fitness more generally.

4.4. The Unstoppable: Misty Copeland

Proving that fitness has no bounds, Misty Copeland, the first Black female principal dancer in the 75-year history of the American Ballet Theater, has orchestrated a dramatic shift in the fitness industry's perception. Ballet, traditionally overshadowed by more conventional forms of exercise, is now gaining immense popularity due to Copeland's towering influence across different social media platforms. By propelling ballet into mainstream fitness, she has managed to spark a unique connection between art and fitness. Her regular posts detailing rigorous practices, coupled with insightful diet tips and inspiring personal anecdotes, inspire millions to harness their inner strength and embrace newfound fitness passions.

These influential women represent an ever-widening spectrum of fitness avenues. Through their daring forays into uncharted territories, they have managed to redefine the fitness landscape. Their approach to promoting a wholesome understanding of fitness, body autonomy, self-care, and resilience amidst obstacles is gradually deconstructing traditional notions of femininity and sport, consequently inspiring a fresh wave of gender-neutral fitness perspectives.

Moreover, what makes these women truly influential is their ability to leverage digital platforms to amplify their messages. With unique strategies, ranging from behind-the-scenes training glimpses to nutritional insights, inclusive community building, or personalized workout challenges, they foster highly engaged digital communities. They not only influence fitness trends, but also catalyze tangible changes in their followers' lifestyles, making healthy living more attainable than ever before.

Each story is a testament to their trailblazing spirit, a powerful reminder of the infinite possibilities that lie within the realm of dedication and persistence. A look at their journeys reveals much more than their fitness prowess; it underlines the element of humanity that binds us all together in the pursuit of our passions and dreams. To sum it up, these women have become leading light houses in the vast sea of fitness, guiding the way by being both enduring symbols of strength and powerful influencers driving transformative changes in every corner of the world. Whether you are at the beginning of your fitness journey, or an experienced athlete seeking inspiration, these profiles offer universal value, pushing the paradigm of what's possible in the ever-evolving realm of fitness. You might just find that in leaping together, we can go farther and reach higher.

Chapter 5. Challenging Norms: The Role of Women in Reinventing Fitness

The voyeur typically beholds a vista teeming with women breaking barriers, making uplifting alterations in the fitness industry - an arena that was once a dominion restrained for the masculine energy. An amalgamation of raw grit, perseverance, unabashed audacity, and sheer resilience has catalyzed a meteoric upheaval in the fitness ecosystem. It is a sight that evokes profound respect for the women advocating for change and enforcing new measures of health and fitness.

5.1. An Unscripted Beginning

Setting the stage for this revolution were the women unwilling to confine themselves within societal norms and expectations. They observed, with a discerning eye, the prevailing definitions of 'fitness' - predominantly heralded by their male counterparts - and longed for a shift. While building strength and muscle was considered a 'men's mission', women were expected to solely endeavour for weight loss, aiming for a narrow aesthetic of 'beauty.' The monolithic narrative was doing more harm than good, breeding a culture of obsession rather than wellness.

Delving into the origins, ironically, the fitness industry was deeply rooted in health and well-being. However, societal norms and mass media distorted its essence, transforming it into an image-oriented market catering to a superficial notion of beauty. The impact was detrimental, especially on women, making them victims of societal pressures and expectations. This took a severe toll on mental health, fostering a culture of body shaming and insecurities. It was high time for a paradigm shift, and the pioneers stepped ahead to redefine standards and challenge norms.

5.2. The Bend Towards Whole-Body Wellness and Strength

A new wave of fitness enthusiasts and trainers emerged, women who were vehement about altering the archaic norms. Fitness was no longer confined to crude, weight-dominated goals. The objective ventured away from 'being skinny' to fostering strength, endurance, flexibility, and overall well-being.

This change begged a deeper understanding of the human body, its needs and capabilities. Instead of adhering to the single narrative of losing weight, trainers began to explore various modalities of movement, and understanding of nutrition, promoting the importance of functional training, and advocating for the mental wellbeing intricately linked to one's physical health. The transformation was gradual but palpable, influencing many along the way.

5.3. Encouraging Diversity in Fitness

Simultaneously, the fitness industry held a mirror to itself, acknowledging the disappointing lack of diversity in its portrayal of health and wellness. The predominant image of "fitness" was often a lean, sculpted white woman. However, reality painted a different picture. Fitness wasn't a one-size-fits-all; it embraced a plethora of body types, ethnicities, ages, and physical capabilities.

The industry began to witness an influx of real people with real stories - women of color, curvy women, older women, women with physical disabilities - all going against the grain to contribute towards a more holistic representation in fitness. This exercise in inclusivity was not just beneficial but necessary, fuelling self-confidence and promoting the acceptance of various body types as fit and healthy.

5.4. Seekers of Change: Women Fitness Influencers

A higher calling to rectify biases pushed women fitness influencers to the forefront. Equipped with tenacity and steeled resolve, they were the embodiment of strength, irrespective of their physical shape and size. They embraced themselves for who they were, adorning their imperfections, their struggles, and their journeys with pride. They perpetuated the concept that fitness is about personal growth, self-love, and self-care.

They leveraged social media platforms to enlighten, widen perspectives and challenge stereotypes. With each Instagram video and YouTube tutorial, they were slowly but steadily revolutionizing the fitness industry, while encouraging hundreds of thousands of followers to look beyond body image and embrace fitness for well-being.

5.5. Shifting Attitude: Body Positivity in Fitness

The insurgence of body positivity in fitness was a breath of fresh air. The notion that all bodies are beautiful, desirable, and, more importantly, capable was largely preached and practiced. Women were taught to appreciate their bodies, irrespective of the societal definitions of 'perfect' or 'beautiful.

This was a potent tool in the industry's arsenal against body shaming and unhealthy self-image. It invited acceptance and celebrated diversity, a tangible shift from the overarching stigmatization and judgment of the past. The energy of body positivity was forceful, empowering women to dismiss external validation and look inward for strength and acceptance.

5.6. The Melting Pot: Women-led Fitness Startups

The causes heralded by these brave women led to a boom in women-led fitness startups. These businesses strived to cultivate environments that were not only conducive to physical transformation but also fostered a sense of belonging and community. They moved beyond the constraints of conventional gyms and offered innovative solutions that resonated with the diverse needs of women. From fitness mobile applications to well-being coaching sessions, personalized workout regimens to democratic fitness-wear innovations, these startups epitomized the evolving demands of the health-conscious society.

In this competitive landscape, the fitness industry's future seems to rest in the capable hands of these women entrepreneurs who triumphantly negotiate societal norms while steadfastly honoring their commitment to promoting health and wellness in their unique, ground-breaking ways.

The relevance and impact of women in the fitness industry have never been more strikingly apparent as they collectively redefine established norms and set new benchmarks. Challenging the status quo, they're on an unparalleled trajectory, valiantly rebuilding the fitness paradigm. Their stories invigorate, inspiring many to view fitness not just as an aesthetic goal but as a path towards self-empowerment and global change. Indeed, the face of fitness has drastically changed and, thanks to these women, continues to evolve organically towards balance and inclusivity.

Chapter 6. Social Media and Fitness: The New Arena for Influence

Social media has irrefutably become a new domain where fitness finds its firm footing. This platform teems with the profound influence of women, who with their inspiring narratives and innovative training approaches, are driving significant changes in our perceptions of health, wellness, and the industry that embodies it.

6.1. The Rise of Fitness Influencers

In the past decade, we have seen a remarkable increase in the number of fitness influencers on prominent social media platforms like Instagram, YouTube, and Facebook. These individuals, particularly women, leverage the power of their personal fitness journeys to inspire and guide millions of people worldwide.

Fitness influencers have become a driving force for change, breaking away from the cookie-cutter, unhealthy ideals of beauty and turning attention towards strength, endurance, and holistic well-being. The key to their influence is authenticity; their followers gravitate towards the relatability of their journey - the successes, the setbacks, the sweat, and the grit. This realness and vulnerability create a more robust, meaningful connection where followers feel seen, included, and motivated.

Women fitness influencers demonstrate a range of fitness realms such as weightlifting, yoga, dance, aerobics, and body positivity, thus providing a smorgasbord of diverse personalities and fitness types for their followers to draw inspiration from. These platforms allow them to lead by example, showcasing the beauty and strength of their resilience, their bodies, and their unyielding spirit.

6.2. Fitness Advice and User Engagement

Leveraging the power of hashtags for cohort formation, blogs for sharing detailed experiences, and live videos for real-time interaction, these influencers cultivate an environment where fitness advice transcends the standard 'one size fits all.' Each influencer, in their style, provides advice ranging from workout routines and meal plans, to mental health discussions and body confidence.

Engagement is fundamental to the robustness of social media influence. Influencers kickstart conversations, challenge their followers with hashtags, and encourage the sharing of personal fitness journeys. They unfailingly respond to queries and comments, breaching the digital divide and ensuring a sense of community respect and camaraderie. This engagement creates a sense of accountability and motivates followers to make positive changes.

6.3. The Marriage of Fitness and Entrepreneurship

The surging popularity of fitness influencers has paved the way towards profitable entrepreneurial ventures. With effective personal branding, they harp on their influence to collaborate with fitness and wellness brands for sponsored posts, merchandise creation, and event partnerships. Some influencers have propelled their influence to launch their own fitness-related startups, offering online workout programs, fitness clothing lines, healthy meal delivery services, and even fitness-focused mobile applications.

This synergy between fitness and entrepreneurship is not only lucrative for the influencers but also shapes the direction of the fitness industry. Misinformation is given a reality check with facts backed by influencers whose years of personal experience and professional fitness training paves the way for honest, effective, and safe fitness advice.

6.4. The Double-edged Sword of Influence

Yet, like all swords, social media influence is double-edged. While it promulgates positive fitness ideals, it can also foster an unhealthy comparison, leading to adverse mental and physical health effects. As consumers of social media, it is vital to admire and draw inspiration but not compare oneself unfavorably. Influencers, too, strive to regularly remind their followers of the same, promoting responsible content consumption.

In the capacious world of social media, the fitness industry has found a powerful ally. Its influence in amplifying women's voices is undeniable, as is its vital role in promoting a more diverse and inclusive portrayal of fitness. By fostering a sense of community, shaping new fitness norms, and bringing momentum to fitness entrepreneurship, it continues to revolutionize the fitness landscape and the portrayal of women within it. Embracing its potential and navigating its challenges, women influencers have indeed transformed this into a new arena for influence.

Chapter 7. Women-led Fitness Startups: Reshaping the Business Landscape

In an era of rapidly evolving fitness trends and reshaping of the wellness industry, women entrepreneurs have emerged as driving forces in introducing innovative fitness startups. The focus of these business endeavors consistently tends towards inclusivity, diversity, and shifting societal perceptions of fitness and health.

7.1. Harnessing the Power of Tech in Fitness

One avenue through which fitness has been revolutionarily redefined is the integration of technology. From fitness apps to wearable gadgets promoting wellness and health, several women have utilized tech innovation to encourage a holistic approach to fitness. Wearable technology has emerged as a major trend in recent years with startups like Bellabeat, headed by Urška Sršen, rising to global acclaim.

Bellabeat, co-founded by Sršen integrates wellness and mindfulness into everyday life using smart jewelry that tracks women's health, stress levels, sleep patterns, and menstrual cycles. The success of Bellabeat confirms that the integration of technology with fitness is not merely a passing fad, but is here to stay, signaling vast opportunities for future entrepreneurs.

Zova, another notable women-led fitness tech startup by Melbourne-based entrepreneur Tanya McCullough and celebrity personal trainer Vix Burdon, provides workouts, mindfulness sessions, sleep tools, and health courses. Tailored for women, by women, the Zova venture imposes technology as a bridging tool promoting the message that fitness is not confined to traditional gym spaces but can be woven seamlessly into our daily routines.

7.2. Shattering Glass Ceilings in the Fitness Business

The fitness industry historically has been male-dominated, presenting numerous challenges for women. However, powerhouse women entrepreneurs have continually defied these obstacles, shattering glass ceilings and paving the way for future female stars in the fitness business.

For instance, Payal Kadakia's ClassPass, a monthly subscription service providing access to different fitness classes around the world, is a prime example. Despite initial setbacks, Kadakia's perseverance and commitment to her vision resulted in ClassPass becoming a unicorn startup valued at over 1 billion dollars, a testament to the game-changing impact women are making on the fitness industry.

Similarly, Emily-Clare Hill and Kat Farrants, the forces behind Movement for Modern Life, a UK-based online yoga platform, symbolize the potential that arises when entrepreneurial creativity meets personal passion for fitness. Their venture, operating on a subscription-based model, has successfully demonstrated how technology can be leveraged to make yoga and mindfulness accessible to a wide user base, irrespective of geographic location or accessibility constraints.

7.3. Embracing Diversity and Inclusion in Fitness

A prominent aspect of the revolution spearheaded by women fitness entrepreneurs is the emphasis on diversity and inclusion. These entrepreneurs are striving to create fitness environments that welcome, embrace, and celebrate all body types, fitness levels, and backgrounds.

One such venture is The Underbelly, a yoga space founded by plus-size yogi Jessamyn Stanley. Stanley, a vocal advocate of body positivity, extends her mission into her venture, promoting inclusivity and acceptance in the fitness world. Her platform provides online yoga classes that are genuinely inclusive and aims to redefine beauty norms in the fitness industry.

In a similar vein, Radha Agrawal's Daybreaker, an early morning dance movement in cities around the world, is an excellent example of a fitness venture that champions community spirit, joy, and inclusivity. Daybreaker hosts sober rave parties in the morning, uniting diverse crowds and pushing the bounds of what's traditionally classified as 'fitness'.

The success, influence, and impact of these businesses underscore the seismic shift in the fitness landscape led by women entrepreneurs. Fueled by a steadfast commitment to engender positive change and an unwavering belief in their vision, these women are redefining fitness on their terms and reshaping the business landscape. This points to an encouraging trend of deep-seated change rooted in inclusivity, technological innovation, and body positivity. Thus, the power of these women-led fitness startups extends far beyond the realm of fitness and penetrates into societal norms, values, and behaviors.

As we look to the future, it's exciting to envision what new innovations will arise through the continued increased participation and leadership of women in the fitness industry. The potential for growth and change is expansive, and these pioneering women entrepreneurs provide a roadmap for how to innovate, inspire, and showcase true power in the world of fitness business.

Chapter 8. Body Positivity in Fitness: The Emerging Trend

The focus of the fitness industry is intuitively shifting, embracing a multi-dimensional model that reframes the meaning of health, beauty, and strength. Body positivity is not merely an emerging trend but is swiftly evolving into the norm, a critical stance against traditional, narrow standards of beauty and fitness. This chapter delves deeply into this seachange, highlighting key figures and moments in the transition to a more inclusive fitness industry.

8.1. Body Positivity: A Paradigm Shift in Fitness

Body positivity, at its core, is the belief that all bodies, regardless of shape, size, age, ethnicity or physical capabilities, are worthy of acceptance and respect. This idea runs counter to the commonly held norms in fitness, which have historically celebrated slim, toned bodies as the epitome of health and attractiveness. However, a growing number of women leaders in the fitness industry vehemently challenge this status quo, advocating for a broader spectrum of representation and diversity that truly captures the diversity of the global population.

Body positivity is revolutionizing fitness in unprecedented ways. It is creating new dialogues and altering perceptions, accepting diversity and inclusivity as fundamental tenets of fitness. It is a revolt against body shaming, promoting self-love and acceptance instead. The shift provides a much-needed balance to universal fitness ideals while preserving the essential goal of health and wellbeing.

8.2. Advocates of Change: Bringing Body Positivity to Fitness

A host of influential women have taken the center stage by representing a myriad of body types in the fitness world. They are actively challenging the fitness industry's ingrained beauty standards, calling for recognition of all body types.

A notable figure in this surge of body positivity is Jessamyn Stanley, an influential yoga teacher, and body positivity advocate. A plus-sized African American woman, Stanley openly defies traditional norms about who can be active, healthy, and engaged in wellbeing pursuits. Through her Instagram presence and app, "The Underbelly Yoga," Stanley inspires people worldwide to reclaim their self-confidence and peace, irrespective of their body shape or size.

Another inspiring influencer is Louise Green, an award-winning fitness trainer and author of "Big Fit Girl." Green is vocal about mobilizing the fitness industry toward inclusivity and diversity. In her book, she empowers plus-sized women to partake in fitness without any constraints of societal judgment or prejudice, redefining what it means to be an athlete or 'fit'.

8.3. The Impact of Social Media on the Body Positivity Movement

Social media has been a game-changer in promoting body-positive fitness. Platforms such as Instagram and YouTube foster dialogues and enable fitness influencers to reach out to millions. Hashtags like #bopo (short for body positive) and #bodyliberation have connected people across the globe, encouraging them to share their unique fitness journeys.

Women fitness leaders harness the power of social media, posting workout routines, tips, and motivational content without airbrushing or sugarcoating the realities of diverse bodies. These authentic posts resonate with a wide audience, affirming that fitness isn't a one-size-fits-all concept. Instead, it's a journey unique to each individual, to be pursued at their pace, style, and comfort.

8.4. Implications and Lessons

The body positivity movement signals a seismic shift in the fitness industry, pushing it towards a more inclusive and empathetic space that raises voices against body-shaming and unrealistic beauty standards. Fitness companies and marketers are also compelled to adopt a more diversified image highlighting bodies of all types and sizes.

While the movement has come a long way in transforming the narrative around fitness and beauty, it still has a distance to go. Everyone involved in the fitness industry, from trainers to entrepreneurs to consumers, must continue to champion inclusivity and the dismantling of harmful stereotypes.

To sum up, the body positivity trend in fitness is an inspiring force that advocates for the respect, acceptance, diversification, and inclusion of all body types. With strong women influencers leading the change, the fitness industry is undoubtedly on its way towards wholesale transformation, one that truly embodies wellness for all.

Chapter 9. Innovation in Workouts: How Women Trainers Are Leading the Way

As we wade more profoundly into the age of innovation and creative thinking, a remarkable transition is visible within the fitness industry. Specifically, the accolades must be given to the influential women at the forefront of this revolution. These dynamic trainers and fitness influencers, powered by unconventional thinking and determination to make faces shine with sweat and joy simultaneously, are daring to transform the traditional narrative. They are not just reinventing how we workout but redefining the boundaries, perceived capabilities, and approaches to fitness.

9.1. Reimagining Traditional Fitness Forms

One striking trend these women are embracing involves the reimagining of traditional fitness forms. Boxing, for instance, has evolved beyond its stereotypical, testosterone-fueled environment. Placing a firm emphasis on empowering all individuals rather than just highlighting aggression, many remarkable women trainers are integrating boxing with other fitness techniques to create unique, hybrid workouts. A similar transformation is seen with yoga, climbing, and even weightlifting, which are being reshaped into diverse, inclusive, and innovative variations.

As an illustrative example, consider the emergence of hybrid yoga forms that blend ancient yoga practices with modern fitness approaches such as pilates, weightlifting, and even dance. Trainers are meticulously combining movement patterns derived from varying disciplines to create comprehensive workouts that challenge norms and keep engagement high. These imaginative fusion programs help participants break away from monotonous routines, offering an enticing freshness to keep you motivated on your fitness journey.

9.2. The Invention of New Workout Styles

You'll also find women trainers leading the invention of entirely new workout styles. The booming popularity of high-intensity interval training (HIIT) programs, the Tabata method, or the recent POUND – Rockout Workout, which combines cardio, strength training with rhythmic movements using lightly-weighted drumsticks, exemplifies the creative genius of women in the fitness industry.

These innovative routines, often built on scientific foundations of exercise physiology, are being adapted to not only cater to the diverse needs of fitness seekers but also mold the workouts into brief, intense, and effective packages. They encapsulate the fast pace of our lives while still focusing on holistic development, challenging the physical, mental, and emotional fortitude of participants.

9.3. Embracing Technology

We must underscore the role of women trainers in embracing and implementing technology into fitness programs. From wearable technology, AI-powered fitness apps, virtual reality-based training to creating sophisticated online platforms, technology has become a permanent resident of the fitness realm, thanks to these forward-thinking women.

Innovative technology incorporation has allowed for personalized workout plans, real-time tracking, and instant feedback, enhancing goal setting, motivation, and outcomes. It has also democratized fitness, making it accessible, customizable, and interactive, shattering the geographical and time barriers that once limited many.

9.4. Sustainability in Fitness

Interestingly, an essential trope of innovative workouts led by women trainers has been sustainability. Recognizing the impact of human actions on the environment, many trainers and fitness organizations, driven by women, are promoting environmentally conscious fitness practices. These include open-air group fitness programs, use of eco-friendly fitness gears, encouraging sustainable diets, and endorsing energy-saving methods in fitness facilities. In essence, they are widening the realm of fitness, intertwining it with global environmental issues, propagating an ethos of world wellness along with personal wellness — a testament to the holistic, comprehensive vision of these women fitness leaders.

9.5. Conclusion

In essence, women trainers are at the forefront of the evolving landscape of the fitness industry, driven by their penchant for innovation, community-building, inclusivity, and a mind-body wellness focus. Their contributions extend beyond concocting effective, engaging workout programs. They are redefining concepts of strength, encouraging positive body image, promoting health at various levels, and leveraging technology and sustainability.

What's more, these are only the heralds of even more exciting innovations to come, as women continue to stretch the echelons of the fitness industry. By cultivating an environment conducive to creativity, adaptation, and change, they are ensuring that fitness remains an accessible, diverse, and empowering journey for everyone. Reflecting on their transformative impact only amplifies the anticipation for what lies ahead in the realm of fitness. The curtain has just risen, and the stage is set for a spectacle that inspires, motivates, and, most importantly, empowers.

Chapter 10. From Global to Grassroots: The Impact of Fitness Influencers on Communities

The advent of social media has allowed fitness influencers to spread their knowledge and fitness journeys from global platforms to grassroots communities. These women, with their empowering stories of fitness transformation, are not merely broadcasting their exercises and diet tips, but are also impacting communities by invigorating a radical shift in the way fitness is perceived and practiced at the ground level.

10.1. Social Media: The Instantaneous Bridge

An important aspect of how women fitness influencers are imparting change is through leveraging social media platforms. platforms like Instagram, YouTube, TikTok, and Facebook have emerged as compelling vehicles of communication, offering an instantaneous bridge between these fitness influencers and the global population. Each post these influencers share—whether it be a workout routine, inspirational quote, dietary advice, or an anecdote from their personal life—has the potential to reach millions of people across continents, thereby sparking conversations and promoting active engagement within diverse communities.

Every comment thread or shared post triggers interactions that bring together people from different walks of life. People who may have previously been marginalized or felt invisible in the global fitness narrative now have a platform to engage, to ask questions, to debate, and most importantly, to learn. Thus, the social media engagement driven by these fitness influencers has had a domino effect, reaching from high-rise condos in bustling cities to quiet suburban homes and even to rural communities with limited resources.

10.2. Inspiring Local Fitness Movements

While being relatable to a global audience is important, many fitness influencers have also tapped into the potential of grassroots movements. There has been a noticeable trend wherein these influencers organize locally-targeted campaigns, marathons, yoga sessions, and boot camps in diverse locations around the world. The aim is to physically reach out to members of the community, motivating them to shake off their inhibitions and take an active leap towards fitness.

Such sessions are more than mere exercise gatherings; they also serve as a platform for personal interaction, both with the influencer and among attendees. These events often end up creating strong local communities that continue to support and drive each other towards fitness goals long after the initial influencer-led session has concluded. Thus, these grassroots fitness movements serve a dual role - promoting physical health and nurturing community bonds, demonstrating that fitness is as much a group endeavor as an individual journey.

10.3. Channeling the Power of Storytelling

Another powerful tool in the hands of these influencers is the art of storytelling. Fitness influencers often share deeply personal journeys of struggle, failure, and subsequent success, making it easier for individuals to connect and find inspiration. The stories may range from overcoming a challenging health condition, fighting oppressive societal norms, or embracing body positivity. These narratives broaden the conversation around fitness, making it more accessible and inclusive.

In their storytelling, women fitness influencers reinforce the idea that fitness is not merely a physical state but an all-encompassing journey of mental, emotional, and spiritual well-being. Moreover, they underscore that fitness is not a cookie-cutter concept; it's a unique journey for each individual. These compelling narratives inspire individuals to craft their own fitness journeys and share their experiences, validating the ebb and flow of the fitness voyage.

10.4. From Online Algorithms to Real-Life Altruism

While their impact online is significant, many fitness influencers extend their influence beyond the world of likes, shares, and comments. They delve into the tangible world through charity programs, empowerment workshops, and mentorship initiatives. They practice what they preach by investing their time and resources into real-world exercises of fitness and community-building, which often go unnoticed in their public profiles.

These influencers understand the value of a holistic approach to fitness, one that encourages a balance between physical strength, mental wellness, and community connection. By stirring these waves of change at the grassroots level, they're essentially revolutionizing the narrative of fitness from being a niche, exclusive domain to an inclusive, hospitable community for all.

In conclusion, women fitness influencers are making an indelible impact, right from global platforms to grassroots communities. From reshaping the conversation around fitness to nurturing local fitness communities and pushing for holistic wellness, they are fundamentally transforming the fitness landscape. And with every story shared, every workshop conducted, every campaign launched, they are empowering individuals around the world to redefine their fitness ideals and reclaim their personal power. We stand on the cusp of a Fitness Revolution, and at its forefront are women influencers daring to disrupt, inspire, and lead.

Chapter 11. Looking Forward: The Future of the Fitness Industry

As we navigate our way into the future, we stand at the precipice of a groundswell - a shifting tidal wave in the fitness industry that is guided, carved, and redefined by women influencers. Women, armed with the dual tools of knowledge and passion, are paving new paths, driving innovation, birthing the transformation of fitness practices, and re-orienting societal perception towards body positivity and holistic well-being.

11.1. The Change Makers: Trends Set by Women in Fitness

Central to this evolution are the trendsetting fitness influencers, who are pushing boundaries, embracing diversity, and highlighting the importance of mental strength alongside physical health. The science of fitness is being democratized and disseminated through blogs, vlogs, podcasts, livestreamed workout sessions and more. The propagators have shifted from hitherto male-centric fitness studios to everyday women who represent a broader spectrum of society, demystifying fitness and making it accessible to all.

Women influencers are shedding light on the connection between mental wellness and physical fitness, promoting practices such as mindfulness and yoga that stress on the importance of aligning the body, mind, and spirit. Furthermore, they are expanding our understanding of fitness to consider internal health markers instead of mere outward appearance, disrupting the traditional narrative of fitness.

Moreover, influencers are pushing the boundaries of traditional training methods by popularizing innovative workout trends. Some of these include HIIT (High-Intensity Interval Training), Functional Training, and Body Weight Training. Such concepts break away from the restrictive nature of gym-based bodybuilding and offer more flexibility, ensuring a wider outreach as individuals can practice these anywhere, even at home.

11.2. The Evolution of Fitness Entrepreneurship

Women's influence extends beyond setting trends - they are also impacting the business of fitness. Fitness startups, led by powerful women entrepreneurs, are growing rapidly, bringing forward fresh business models that prioritize customer health and wellness. They are introducing biohacking, nutrient-dense food services, personalized fitness and meal planning applications, accessible gym equipment, wearable fitness tech, and more.

Strikingly, women entrepreneurs are taking inclusive steps to ensure their services cater to a diverse range of clientele, including those typically underserved by the fitness industry such as older adults or individuals with specific health issues. In doing so, they are making fitness a more inclusive landscape.

11.3. The Significance of Social Media in Future Fitness

As we peer into the future, we see social media continuing to play a pivotal role across the fitness industry. Women influencers are leveraging social media platforms such as Instagram, YouTube, and TikTok to spread healthier body narratives and destigmatize various body forms. The growing trend of 'Insta Fit' celebrates real, unedited bodies and emphasizes the importance of feeling good over looking good. Influencers also showcase holistic health, advocating for everyday women to take control of their wellness journeys and to engage in fitness activities that bring joy alongside health benefits.

Women influencers are also shaping the tonality of fitness conversations on social media. They are increasingly focusing on empowerment, self-love, perseverance, and resilience, over the antiquated measure of gauging fitness by appearances. This overall narrative shift, carried forward by women influencers, is expected to radically shape the future discourse and understanding of fitness.

11.4. The Forecast: Direction of Women-Led Fitness Revolution

As we look to the future, we see an industry that is inclusive, authentic, and concerned with overall wellness. The movement, driven by women influencers, pushes the pendulum away from punitive, unrealistic body standards towards diverse, holistic, body-positive fitness ideals. It emphasizes the need for fitness to retain its essence - to be about health, strength,, resilience, balance - and not just an aesthetically-driven pursuit.

Driven by technology, we foresee an era of personalized fitness where individual data will drive optimized training regimens. The advent of AI trainers, VR workouts, and biometric wearable technology, championed by women entrepreneurs, points towards a dynamically evolving fitness landscape rich with potential.

However, the future is not without its challenges. There will be continued efforts needed to address issues of diversity and inclusion in all aspects of fitness, and to systematically dismantle deep-seated body shaming narratives. But given the concerted resolve echoed by women influencers and entrepreneurs in the fitness industry, we anticipate a sustained revolution that redefines the fitness industry in an egalitarian, inclusive, and wellness-oriented manner.

In summary, the future of the fitness industry showcases a promising narrative, one that's driven by women influencers and entrepreneurs globally. This paradigm shift, shaped by innovative concepts, technological advancements, and based on the bedrock of inclusivity, body positivity and holistic well-being, ushers us into a new era of fitness, one that's poised to transform societal perceptions and attitudes on an unprecedented scale.